For Women Only

THE
CLITORIS

(How many do you actually have?)

Experience multiple orgasms,
anywhere,
anytime,
without even hopping into bed.

by The Love Doctor

For Women Only
THE CLITORIS
(How many do you actually have?)
Experience multiple orgasms, anywhere, anytime, without even hopping into bed.
All Rights Reserved.
Copyright © 2019 The Love Doctor
v1.0

THE LOVE DOCTOR

ISBN: 978-0-578-21513-6

PRINTED IN THE UNITED STATES OF AMERICA

TABLE OF CONTENTS

INTRODUCTION

THIS HANDBOOK IS inspired by the discoveries created by the true love and passion between the author and his wife. We are not sex maniacs, but because of the depth of our relationship, the unconditional love we have for each other, there is a true passion that we share for each other which creates this burning desire to be affectionate towards each other 24 hours a day, 365 days a year.

Hopefully, you will find this handbook helpful in your relationship with your significant other, and it will bring you both orgasmic pleasures the likes of which you never dreamed possible.

For Women Only

Chapter One

WHAT IS THE CLITORIS?

I KNOW THAT you are very anxious to find out what this writer is wanting to disclose to you, but it is necessary to define the clitoris. For this purpose I am borrowing a description of the clitoris from Mr. Tim Taylor, Anatomy and Physiology Instructor, which I found at Innerbody.com and which is for educational purposes only and should not be taken as expert advice.

The clitoris is a small projection of erectile tissue in the vulva of the female reproductive system. It contains thousands of nerve endings that make it an extremely sensitive organ. Touch stimulation of the nerve endings in the clitoris produces sensations of sexual pleasure, and if properly massaged can produce incredible, uncontrollable female orgasms.

The clitoris is located within the vulva at the anterior intersection of the labia minora. It is vaguely cylindrical in shape and usually just a centimeter or two in length, although its size may vary greatly in individuals. The prepuce, or hood of the clitoris, is a small fold of skin that covers and protects the clitoris anteriorly; the labia majora and the labia minora surround and protect it in all other directions.

The clitoris can be divided into three major regions: glans, body, and crura.

Under the surface of the skin, two legs of erectile tissue known as the crura fan out to support the exterior and attach to the underlying tissues. Extending from the crura is the body, the main cylindrical region of the clitoris, which contains two columns of the erectile tissue. Blood filling the hollow chambers of the erectile tissue allows the clitoris to grow in size and harden during sexual stimulation.

Finally, the glans forms the pointed tip of the clitoris extending outward from the body and beyond the prepuce that covers the rest of the clitoris.

Thousands of touch- and pressure-sensitive nerve endings are found throughout the clitoris. Nerve endings in the body and glans are sensitive to direct touch and pressure stimulation from outside of the body, while nerve endings of the crus are sensitive to stimulation from within the vagina. The stimulation of the clitoris' nerve endings is responsible for the majority of sexual pleasure and sensation of the female body.

Now that you have had the opportunity to read and hopefully understand the physical description of the clitoris and its function during sexual activity, it is time to move to the next chapters, which will attempt to explain to you just how many clitorises one female can actually have, and how they can be found. This will give you an understanding of this subject, and hopefully various ways through which you will experience multiple orgasms—the likes of which you never dreamed possible!!!!

Chapter Two

PHYSICAL RELEASE

PHYSICAL RELEASE CAN be achieved in only a few ways and is nothing more than what could be described as "Climax." Climax occurs as a result of a sufficient amount of stimulation that can be derived from visual stimuli (such as watching others engage in sexual activity), masturbation (self-administered activity), and casual sexual activity with others of the same or opposite sex.

Climax, being strictly physical in nature, cannot compare to the experience of obtaining complete and total Orgasms. If and when you are fortunate enough to experience complete and total orgasms, you will understand the difference and you will be amongst the luckiest people in the world. This unbelievable physical and emotional release cannot be realized by any of the above-described methods of Climax.

Chapter Three

PASSION

FOR OUR PURPOSES, Passion can easily be described as "an uncontrollable feeling of intense enthusiasm or compelling desire towards someone."

Passion for someone is only instilled in us when we are truly in love with another. For us to experience True Love with our partner in life, the following components must exist between both parties: truth, communication, trust, respect, and an undying faith in and unconditional commitment to each other.

If you are fortunate enough to have all of these exist in your relationship, then your passion for each other will bring you to experience the highest of highs in your relationship and the sensitivities in your physical and emotional being. You will discover new heights and awareness of all of your sensitivities.

Chapter Four

CLITORIS IN YOUR HANDS

WHEN YOU SHARE the mutual passion discussed previously with your life partner, you will find many areas of your body that physically and emotionally provide such incredible sensations that you will reach orgasms the likes of which you have never before experienced.

These orgasms can happen anytime and anywhere.

Holding hands with your life partner is a natural and frequent occurrence. The insides of your palm and your fingertips contain thousands of nerve endings, just as your clitoris does. Gentle touching of these areas of your palm while holding hands stimulates all of these nerve endings, which can and do lead to uncontrollable emotional and physical orgasms that will take you by surprise and can happen anywhere. Therefore you must each be cautious not to let this happen whenever you are in public or mixed company.

The first time this happened between my wife and me, before we were married, we were on a road trip. Being very deeply in love with each other, we were holding hands while I was driving. I was also gently touching the inside of her palm with my index finger, when suddenly she seemed to go into uncontrollable convulsions. I immediately pulled the car over to the side of the road and ran around to open her door. I did not recognize what was happening to her. When I opened her door, she immediately put her arms around me, and at that precise moment I knew she was having a massive orgasm. I held her as tight as I could and kissed her lips passionately as she continued to orgasm over and over. What an experience for both of us. To think that I could give her such pleasure simply by touching her palm was as satisfying for me as it was for her. Truly, the palm of her hand acted as a clitoris neither of us knew she had.

There have been other times when this has accidently happened to us, such as being in one of our favorite restaurants, when my wife suddenly excused herself and went to the ladies' room, where her orgasm peaked without any further stimulation. We continue to do our best to avoid this happening in public places, but because of the depth of our love for each other sometimes it just happens.

I suggest you try this with your loved one, but make sure you're not anywhere in public or in the presence of others.

Chapter Five

CLITORIS IN YOUR MOUTH

KISSING IS QUITE a normal happening between lovers. But when the passion between two lovers is so strong, a French kiss alone can lead to a massive orgasm. Like the clitoris, the tongue has thousands of nerve endings. The stimulation of your tongue by your life partner, coupled with the closeness of your bodies, clothed or not, can cause you to orgasm without any other form of stimulation.

When my wife and I were first dating, we did not share a French kiss for the first month or so. She and I lived in the same neighborhood, and one night when I was walking her to her car, I went to kiss her good night and we ended up having our first French kiss. It wasn't a long kiss, but she immediately got in her car and drove home. I did not learn until after we were married that the reason she departed so quickly was because she was having an orgasm right there in my driveway, and she was embarrassed that I might recognize what was happening to her. Since that time, my wife has had many very strong orgasms just from us sharing a French kiss.

Try it for yourself with your life partner, but be discreet. Not in public or in the presence of others.

Chapter Six

CLITORIS IN YOUR FEET

JUST ABOUT EVERY nerve in your body ends in the bottom of your feet. Unlike any other part of your body, your feet are more sensitive to touch than most people recognize. Think about your last doctor's visit where the doctor tested your reflexes. The doctor gently stroked the bottoms of your feet and your toes reacted by turning down.

Now imagine your life partner gently kissing the bottoms of your feet with their tongue!!! The sensitivity in your feet will cause stimulation to almost every nerve in your body, bringing you to yet another incredible orgasmic experience.

The first time I did this to my wife, we both experienced an incredible orgasm together. Between the sensitivity in her feet and in my tongue, the excitement was uncontrollable.

Needless to say, this activity should be confined to private places, such as the bedroom, or anywhere else in the house as long as the two of you are alone.

Chapter Seven

CLITORIS IN YOUR KNEES

THE BACKS OF your knees are extremely sensitive to the touch. Perhaps you may have noticed this whenever you have had a good massage?

Now picture in your mind your significant other, having finished with your feet, working his way up your calves with his tongue while you are lying on your stomach. The anticipation is building as he gets closer and closer to the backs of your knees. Finally he starts to gently kiss the back of one knee and then begins to massage it with his tongue. The sensation will drive you wild, and within a very short time you will experience yet another explosive, uncontrollable orgasm.

But wait, there's more to come. That was just one knee! What about the other one? It is begging to receive the same attention, and when it does you'd better be ready for it!!! This next orgasm will be twice as intense as the first one.

Chapter Eight

CLITORIS INNER THIGHS

YOU HAVE NOW experienced a minimum of four orgasms the likes of which you have never experienced, and we're just getting started.

Now it's time to discover just how sensitive your inner thighs are. And remember, you have two of those too.

After you've recovered from your orgasms of your feet and knees, it's time to move to one of your inner thighs. So turn over and lie on your back, spread your legs, and let your lover go to work.

Gently he starts kissing your inner thigh with occasional pressure from his teeth. If he happens to have a soft beard, you will experience even more sensitivity. His tongue starts licking and you can barely control yourself. You are moaning, starting to breathe heavily. And then it happens!!! Another explosive orgasm, and just as you are coming to the end of it, he repeats the same activity on the other inner thigh. And just like the second knee, this orgasm is twice as intense as the first one.

My God!!! you are thinking! We started making love an hour ago and already I'm in heaven. I want more, more, more!!!

Chapter Nine

CLITORIS NAVEL

YOU ARE IN ecstasy, and your lover is working his way from your inner thighs towards your abdomen. His tongue now finds your navel and starts to gently massage the inside of it. You gently stroke your fingers through his hair, pulling his head closer and closer as his tongue gently works all around and inside your navel. The sensation becomes overwhelming and you break into another uncontrollable orgasm.

Chapter Ten

CLITORIS ABDOMEN

NOW YOUR LOVER slowly moves to the right side of your lower abdomen. His tongue, lips, and teeth are gently massaging your skin. Finally his mouth reaches your very right side, just above your hip. The sensation of his activity is becoming more and more intense. You are in ecstasy and trying to control your emotions, but it's no use. Your passion for your lover and the incredible sensations of his tenderness give way and you explode into another massive orgasm.

He holds you tightly, pressing his head on your stomach, and as he does, your anticipation starts building as you know that he is heading for your left side to repeat himself. When he reaches your left side you again explode within seconds. How can this be happening? you think to yourself. Stop thinking! Just enjoy and savor the experience!!!

Chapter Eleven

CLITORIS BREASTS

MOST WOMEN ARE very much aware of the sensitivity of their breasts, especially their nipples. Women love to have their lover caress and massage their breasts with their hands. But when your lover gently places his mouth over your nipple, starts massaging it gently with his tongue, and gently bites the erected tip coupled with gentle sucking, the sensation you experience becomes mind blowing. You begin to feel emotional and physical highs and a closeness to your lover that makes you feel you want this to go on forever.

Your lover is so attuned to your reaction that he is purposely taking his time, knowing that by doing so he is bringing you towards yet another massive release. And this is only on one breast! You have another one which, in your mind, you are begging him to go to next. And when he does the sensations and emotions you experience are twice as strong.

After all of the orgasms you have just experienced, you beg your lover for a little rest. He accommodates you and holds you in his arms with your head resting gently on his chest. You can't help yourself because the depth of your love for each other is so strong, so you gently start running your hands over his chest and abdomen. Of course you know that this will arouse him, and you gently move your hands over his rock-hard erection.

This will definitely lead to much, much more!!!!!!

Chapter Twelve

CLITORIS HANDS AND ARMS

THE TWO OF you are caressing each other. He is lying on his back with your head nestled into his shoulder. Your hand has been gently stroking his chest, stomach, and his rock-hard manhood. He gently takes your hand and puts it over his face, your palm covering his mouth. Softly he starts to kiss the inside of your palm. You are tempted to resist, because you know where this will lead and you just don't know if you can handle much more at this time. But he holds it close to his lips with his hand and gently starts to massage the inside of your palm with his tongue. It's not long before the sensation and excitement you are experiencing leads to yet another explosive orgasm.

He turns towards you, pressing his body close to yours, and you can feel his erection right next to your vagina. You pull him even closer as he takes your arm and starts kissing your forearm, moving towards the inside of your elbow. Once there, his kisses and tongue massages take you to a new high in emotional, spiritual, and physical ecstasy. The sensations running through your mind and body make you feel like you never want this to end, and you are doing your best to savor every last second, when without warning it happens!! An orgasm more intense than all of the others you have just experienced.

He's not done! In fact he's just warming up. Now he moves to the inside of your bicep. WOOOOO!!! You never thought this part of your body could be so sensitive! But he's not going to let you have an orgasm here, even though he knows he can make that happen. No, by this time he knows that you are ready, willing, and able to let him go wherever he wants to—and that is exactly what he does.

He takes your arm and gently raises it, exposing your armpit. As he lovingly looks at it he can see how soft and tender it is, and he can't resist. Gently he starts to kiss all around it, and then once he has it soaking in his saliva, he goes to work with his tongue. Your mind is whirling; it's becoming hard to breathe. You know where this is going to take you and you try your best to resist. But it's no use! You explode with another unbelievable orgasm!!!!

Your anticipation is uncontrollable as you know that you have another hand, another arm, and another armpit—and that's exactly where he's going next!!

Chapter Thirteen

CLITORIS NECK

WOW, DOES YOUR lover ever love to kiss your neck. It is such a tender part of your body and has the stimulating fragrance of your favorite perfume. He loves to have his lips and tongue all over it. He loves to suck on it and softly bite it. He knows that it is one of the more sensitive parts of your body, and loving to do all of these things, he knows that he can bring you to even more beautiful and exciting orgasms.

Chapter Fourteen

CLITORIS EARS

EVER HAD YOUR ears massaged by your lover's tongue? Not only are the insides of your ears sensitive to this, but there is added excitement caused by the actual sounds created by his tongue gently massaging the insides of your ears. This very exciting activity does not need to be confined to the bedroom. It can take place in the kitchen, while you're preparing breakfast, lunch, or dinner. You can be sitting in your favorite chair and your mate can quietly come up behind you and start nibbling on your ear, bringing you to an extremely passionate orgasm. If you haven't had this experience, it is highly recommended, as it is just one more physical and emotional activity between you and your significant other that stirs the heart, body, mind, and soul, bringing the two of you ever closer and more deeply in love with each other.

Chapter Fifteen

SUMMATION

IN THE PREVIOUS chapters I have described twenty-four areas of a woman's body that react exactly the same way as a woman's clitoris. Each and every one of these areas has the ability to produce physical and emotional orgasms the likes of which most women have never before experienced.

Some of these sensitive areas of the woman's body can be massaged and kissed outside the privacy of the home, bedroom, or hotel room; however, you need to be very discreet when employing them out in the public world. It could prove very embarrassing for both of you, as you could have totally unexpected emotional and physical orgasms when you least expect them.

When you are in the privacy of your own home it's "NO HOLDS BARRED," and you can experiment with any of these sensitive areas described in this booklet. Bear in mind that you don't have to explore all of these areas in one Lovemaking session, but if you intend to, be prepared for several hours of emotional, physical, and passionate lovemaking that will take you to "ORGASMIC HEAVEN" the likes of which you have never before experienced and will bring you closer to your significant other than you ever dreamed possible.

I hope you find this booklet helpful and suggest that as you experience these sensitive areas of your newfound clitorises, you may also discover other areas of your body that react in the same way.

Always remember that life is a journey of learning new things every day. When it comes to our physical and emotional well-being, there is nothing healthier than the Orgasmic pleasures that can be brought through TRUE, UNCONDITIONAL LOVE!!!!!